THE KIDNEY CHRONICLES

Navigating the Journey to

Optimal Health

Dr. Thomas K. McGlynn

TABLE OF CONTENTS

INTRODUCTION

The kidneys are a pair of relatively tiny yet powerful organs. They are in charge of filtering waste products and excess fluids from your blood, regulating the balance of minerals and fluids in your body, producing hormones that regulate blood pressure and support the production of red blood cells, and a great deal more besides. They are responsible for all of these things and more. Despite the vital role, they play in preserving your overall health, the kidneys often get very little attention until something is seriously wrong with them.

Kidney disease is a developing public health problem that already impacts the lives of millions of people all over the globe. It can produce a wide variety of symptoms, ranging from slight discomfort to life-threatening consequences, and if it is not treated, it may lead to kidney failure. On the other hand, many instances of kidney illness are capable of being properly controlled if they are caught early and given the appropriate treatment.

In this book, we will delve into the intricate world of the kidneys and their functions, the myriad forms of kidney disease and the factors that contribute to their development, and the actions that you can take to ensure your kidneys are in the best possible health and to treat kidney disease if you have it. You will discover helpful information and advice that you can put into practice on these pages, regardless of whether you are a patient, a caregiver, or just someone interested in learning more about this important area of health.

An Explanation of the Kidneys and Their Roles in the Body

The kidneys are two bean-shaped organs that may be found immediately below the ribcage in the center of the back. Each kidney is around the size of a fist and weighs about a half pound on average. In addition to the protection provided by the ribcage, the kidneys are shielded by a layer of fat.

The kidneys' principal job is to remove waste materials and excess fluids from the blood, which are subsequently expelled from the body in the form of urine. Urine is how the kidneys accomplish this task. This process is essential for preserving the body's natural equilibrium of minerals and fluids, as well as for controlling blood pressure and heart rate. In addition, the kidneys are responsible for the generation of hormones that control the creation of red blood cells and contribute to the development of healthy bones.

In addition to acting as filters for waste, the kidneys are responsible for several other critical tasks, including the following:

The kidneys are responsible for the production of the hormone known as renin, which plays a role in the regulation of blood pressure. Renin sends a signal to the blood vessels to constrict when blood pressure is too low, which causes blood pressure to rise.

Erythropoietin is a hormone that promotes the production of red blood cells in the bone marrow. Erythropoietin is produced by the bone marrow.

The kidneys play a role in maintaining a healthy balance of minerals in the body by controlling the levels of sodium, potassium, and phosphorus, among other elements.

Activating vitamin D, the kidneys are responsible for activating vitamin D, which is essential for maintaining healthy bones and a functioning immune system.

Additionally, the kidneys have a degree of their own inherent capacity for self-repair and regeneration. In the event that one of the kidneys is injured, the other kidney is able to compensate and take on more work in order to keep the kidneys' overall function intact.

The kidneys are responsible for a significant portion of the body's general health and well-being maintenance. The prevention of kidney illness and the protection of these crucial organs during their whole lifespan both depend on the patient's ability to keep their kidneys in excellent working order.

The Significance of Preserving Normal Kidney Function at All Costs

It is essential for both general health and lifespan to take care of one's kidneys and keep them in excellent condition. The kidneys are responsible for removing waste and surplus fluids from the body, controlling blood pressure, creating hormones, and maintaining mineral balance. They also play an important role in regulating blood pressure. It is possible for waste products and fluid to build up in the body when the kidneys are not operating correctly, which may lead to a variety of health concerns as well as complications that might possibly be life-threatening.

Keeping Your Kidneys in Good Condition Is Essential for A Number of Reasons, Including the Following:

Preventing Kidney Disease: The prevention of kidney disease is one of the most important reasons to take care of one's kidneys and keep them in good condition. Chronic kidney disease, also known as CKD, is a prevalent disorder that has the potential to be fatal and is associated with a wide variety of symptoms, ranging from slight discomfort to serious damage to internal organs. Keeping your kidneys in excellent condition by making decisions that are favorable to your lifestyle and going in for checkups on a regular basis will help avoid the development of chronic kidney disease (CKD).

Keeping a Healthy Blood Pressure: The kidneys play a crucial role in the regulation of blood pressure, and when they are not functioning properly, blood pressure can become elevated, which can lead to other health problems such as heart disease, stroke, and kidney damage. Maintaining Healthy Blood Pressure, the kidneys play a crucial role in the regulation of blood pressure. It is essential for both the kidneys and the body as a whole to have appropriate blood pressure levels at all times.

Maintaining Bone Health: The kidneys are involved in the activation of vitamin D, which is necessary for maintaining healthy bones and immunological function. Vitamin D is vital for maintaining strong bones. It is particularly important for those who are older to take care of their kidneys since doing so may help avoid bone loss and osteoporosis.

Regulating Electrolyte Balance: The kidneys play a role in maintaining a healthy electrolyte balance in the body by contributing to the regulation of the levels of minerals such as sodium, potassium, and phosphorus. These mineral levels may become unbalanced, which can lead to a variety of health concerns, including muscular weakness, cardiac arrhythmias, and other disorders. This can occur when the kidneys are not working correctly.

Production of Red Blood Cells: The kidneys are responsible for the production of the hormone erythropoietin, which promotes the production of red blood cells in the bone marrow. A healthy supply of red blood cells is necessary for excellent health and energy levels; thus, it is important to take care of one's kidneys so that they remain in good condition.

In conclusion, preserving a healthy kidney is critical for lowering the risk of developing diseases and other difficulties, bolstering overall health and well-being, and achieving and sustaining a high quality of life. The key to preserving excellent kidney health is to get routine checkups, make lifestyle choices that are healthy, and discover any potential issues as early as possible.

CHAPTER 1

Understanding Kidney Disease

A disorder that causes the kidneys to gradually lose function over time is referred to as kidney disease, which is also known as chronic kidney disease (CKD). This may result in a variety of health issues and consequences, including the accumulation of waste products and fluid in the body, as well as a wide range of other health concerns. Kidney illness is a significant public health problem that affects millions of individuals all over the globe. In the United States, it ranks as the ninth largest cause of death overall.

The capacity of your body to clean your blood, filter excess water out of your blood, and assist maintain your blood pressure might be negatively impacted when you have a kidney illness. Additionally, it may interfere with the creation of red blood cells and the metabolism of vitamin D, both of which are essential for maintaining bone health.

You start off with two kidneys when you're born. You may find them on each side of your spine, just above where your waist is.

It is possible for your body to accumulate waste materials as well as fluid when your kidneys are impaired. Because of this, you may have swelling in your ankles, nausea, weakness, disturbed sleep, and shortness of breath. In the absence of therapy, the damage may get more severe, and you may ultimately lose the ability to use your kidneys. That is a major issue, and it may even pose a danger to one's life.

The Role That Your Kidneys Play

Remove waste from your blood after digestion, muscular activity, and exposure to chemicals or pharmaceuticals Kidneys that are healthy do the following:

- Maintain a healthy balance of water and minerals (such as salt, potassium, and phosphorus) in your blood.
- Remove waste from your blood.
- Produce renin, which is used by your body to assist in the management of your blood pressure.
- Produce a substance known as erythropoietin, which causes your body to produce red blood cells.

- Produce an active form of vitamin D, which is required for bone health and a variety of other functions.

There Are a Number of Distinct Forms of Kidney Disease, Including the Following:

An acute injury to the kidneys: This is a rapid and transient loss of kidney function, which is often brought on by an accident or a preexisting health condition.

The most important factors are:

- Direct injury to the kidneys
- Urine accumulation in the kidneys
- Not enough blood flow to the kidneys

These things can occur when you:

• Have a traumatic injury with blood loss, such as in a car accident

• Are dehydrated or your muscle tissue breaks down, sending too much kidney-toxic protein into your bloodstream These things can happen when you:

• Are dehydrated or your muscle tissue breaks down

• You will experience shock as a result of a severe illness known as sepsis.

• Take certain medications or are exposed to certain toxins that directly damage the kidneys

• Have complications during pregnancy, such as eclampsia and preeclampsia

• Have an enlarged prostate or kidney stones that block your urine flow

Chronic Kidney Disease (CKD): is characterized by a gradual and steady decline in kidney function over the course of time. This decline is due to a number of underlying causes. Chronic renal disease is a condition that is characterized by a decline in kidney function that has persisted for more than three months. During the early stages, you may not have any symptoms, but this is the time when it is easiest to treat.

High blood pressure and diabetes, both kinds 1 and 2, are the leading causes of death worldwide. Your kidneys might suffer damage if you have high blood sugar levels for an extended period of time. In addition, high blood pressure causes the blood arteries in your body, especially the ones that provide blood to your kidneys, to get worn down.

Glomerulonephritis: is the collective term for a collection of disorders that affect the kidneys and are characterized by inflammation of the kidney's microcirculation, which ultimately results in kidney damage.

Polycystic Kidney Disease (PKD): often known as PKD, is a hereditary condition that manifests itself as the development of cysts inside the kidneys. This, in turn, may result in the kidneys being progressively damaged and diseased.

Nephrotic Syndrome: a combination of symptoms that develops when the kidneys lose a significant quantity of protein in the urine. This condition is also known as the nephrotic state.

Nephritis: Nephritis is a term that refers to inflammation of the kidneys, which can be caused by a variety of underlying conditions, including infections, autoimmune diseases, and certain medications. This inflammation can be caused by nephritis.

Kidney Stones: Kidney stones are painful ailments that may be caused when tiny, solid deposits of minerals and salts accumulate in the kidneys. These stones can also create obstructions in the urinary canal and give the patient discomfort.

Urinary Tract Infections (UTIs): Urinary tract infections (also known as UTIs) are infections that may develop anywhere in the urinary system, including the kidneys, the bladder, and the urethra. If the infection is not adequately treated, it can cause damage to the kidneys.

It is essential to have a solid understanding of the fact that kidney disease may be brought on by a wide range of underlying conditions, as well as the significance of early diagnosis and appropriate treatment in preventing significant consequences. It is vital to share any symptoms or concerns you may be having with your healthcare practitioner if you are worried about the health of your kidneys.

Symptoms and Diagnosis

The following are the symptoms of kidney disease:

It is possible that kidney illness will not produce any obvious symptoms in its earlier stages. However, as the illness advances, there is a possibility that some symptoms, including the following:

Fatigue and weakness: The buildup of waste materials in the blood might be a contributing factor in the symptoms of fatigue and weakness.

Swelling: Swelling may happen in the face, ankles, and legs when the kidneys are unable to eliminate extra fluid from the body. Swelling can also develop in the legs.

Foamy Urine: A typical symptom of kidney illness is the presence of foamy urine, which may develop if there is an excessive amount of protein in the urine.

Urinating more or less frequently: Alterations in the way the kidneys normally work might lead to an increase or decrease in the number of times per day that a person urinates.

Back or side pain: Pain in the back or the sides is one symptom that may be present when there is an issue with the kidneys or another component of the urinary system.

Nausea and vomiting: Nausea and vomiting are symptoms that may appear if there is an accumulation of waste materials in the blood, which may lead to a sickening sensation throughout the body.

Skin rashes or itching: Rash or itching of the skin is one of the symptoms that may appear if there is a buildup of waste materials in the blood, which is known to irritate the skin.

Diagnosis of Kidney Disease

The process of diagnosing kidney disease often includes a physical exam, testing of blood and urine, and tests of urine. The amounts of creatinine, a waste product that is generally filtered out by the kidneys and is formed as a byproduct of the metabolism of muscle, may be measured using blood testing. An elevated amount of creatinine in the blood may be an indicator of impaired renal function. The quantities of protein and other waste products in the urine, which may also be a symptom of kidney impairment if they are elevated, can be measured using urine testing.

Imaging techniques such as ultrasound, computed tomography (CT), and magnetic resonance imaging (MRI) may also be used to analyze the kidneys and identify any structural abnormalities or issues that may be present.

It is essential to be aware of the possible signs of kidney disease and to address any concerns with your healthcare practitioner. If you have any questions or concerns about your health, you should contact your healthcare provider. In order to avoid more severe issues and to keep one's kidneys in healthy working order, early identification and treatment are very necessary.

Causes as well as Potential Risk Factors

Diseases of the Kidneys Can Be Caused By:

There are several potential contributors to the development of kidney disease, including the following:

High blood pressure: Prolonged exposure to a high blood pressure reading may cause permanent damage to the blood vessels found in the kidneys, which can ultimately result in kidney disease.

Diabetes: High amounts of glucose in the blood over an extended period of time may cause damage to the blood vessels in the kidneys, which can lead to kidney disease.

Glomerulonephritis: Glomerulonephritis is the collective term for a collection of disorders that affect the kidneys and are characterized by inflammation of the kidney's microcirculation, which ultimately results in kidney damage.

Polycystic Kidney Disease (PKD): Polycystic Kidney Disease, often known as PKD, is a hereditary condition that manifests itself as the development of cysts inside the kidneys. This, in turn, may result in the kidneys being progressively damaged and diseased.

Nephrotic Syndrome: Nephrotic syndrome is a combination of symptoms that develops when the kidneys lose a significant quantity of protein in the urine. This condition is also known as the nephrotic state.

Nephritis: Nephritis is a term that refers to inflammation of the kidneys, which can be caused by a variety of underlying conditions, including infections, autoimmune diseases, and certain medications. This inflammation can be caused by nephritis.

Kidney stones: Kidney stones are painful ailments that may be caused when tiny, solid deposits of minerals and salts accumulate in the kidneys. These deposits can lead to obstructions in the urinary canal and give the patient discomfort.

Urinary tract infections (UTIs): Urinary tract infections, often known as UTIs, are infections that may develop anywhere in the urinary system, including the kidneys, the bladder, and the urethra. If the infection is not adequately treated, it can cause damage to the kidneys.

Exposure to drugs and toxins: Some medicines and chemicals, particularly those that are used for a lengthy period of time or at high doses, have the potential to cause harm to the kidneys.

Factors That Increase the Danger of Kidney Disease

There are a number of risk factors that, when combined, may increase the possibility of getting kidney disease. These risk factors, in addition to the primary causes of kidney disease, include the following:

Age: The likelihood of developing kidney disease is proportional to one's age.

Family history: The presence of a history of kidney disease in one's family is associated with an increased chance of developing the ailment.

Ethnicity: People of certain racial and ethnic backgrounds, including African Americans, Native Americans, and Hispanic Americans, have a higher incidence of kidney disease than other groups in the United States.

Cigarette smoking: Cigarette smoking is linked to an increased risk of kidney disease, in addition to an increased risk of many other health concerns.

Obesity: Being overweight or obese may raise a person's chance of developing kidney disease, in addition to the risk of developing other health concerns.

It is important to be aware of your risk for kidney disease and to take steps to reduce your risk. These steps include maintaining a healthy lifestyle, controlling blood pressure and blood sugar levels, and avoiding exposure to drugs and toxins that can cause damage to the kidneys. Knowing your risk and taking steps to reduce your risk are both important.

It is vital to share your worries about your risk for kidney disease with your healthcare professional if you are worried about your likelihood of developing the condition.

Medications Used to Treat Kidney Disease

The stage of kidney disease as well as the underlying cause of the illness will determine how the disease is treated. Changes in lifestyle, like adopting a nutritious diet, maintaining a regular exercise routine, and giving up smoking, may help delay the course of the illness and reduce the risk of problems in the early stages.

It is possible to cure some manifestations of renal disease. These therapies are aimed at reducing the severity of the symptoms, preventing the illness from progressing further, and minimizing the risk of consequences. There is a possibility that some of your kidney function may be restored as a result of your therapy. There is currently no treatment available for chronic renal disease.

What's causing your kidney illness will determine the treatment strategy that you and your physician choose to implement. Even when the underlying cause of your ailment is treated, there is always a possibility that your kidney disease may worsen.

You will need therapy for the end-stage renal disease once your kidneys reach the point where they are unable to process waste on their own.

Medication, such as angiotensin-converting enzyme (ACE) inhibitors or angiotensin receptor blockers (ARBs), may also be recommended in order to assist with the regulation of blood pressure and the protection of the kidneys.

In more severe stages, patients may need kidney transplants or dialysis to maintain their health. Through the use of a machine, the process known as "dialysis" removes waste materials and excess fluid from the patient's blood. During a kidney transplant operation, a healthy kidney is removed from a donor and surgically implanted into the recipient patient.

Avoiding the Development of Kidney Disease

There are a number of measures one may take to assist avoid kidney disease and keep one's kidneys in excellent condition. These measures include the following:

Maintaining a healthy lifestyle: Keeping a healthy lifestyle is accomplished by not smoking, participating in regular physical exercise, consuming a moderate amount of alcohol, and eating balanced food.

Managing other health conditions: This includes lowering blood pressure in those with high blood pressure and reducing blood sugar levels in people who have diabetes.

Drinking plenty of water: Consuming a large quantity of water may assist in the removal of waste products and excess fluids from the body, hence lowering the chance of developing kidney stones.

Getting regular check-ups and kidney function tests: Receiving regular checkups and evaluations of your kidney function: May assist in the early detection of kidney illness and enable fast treatment to be administered, hence reducing the risk of significant consequences.

In conclusion, kidney disease is a severe and rising public health problem; nevertheless, it is possible to avoid and control the condition via early identification, appropriate treatment, and maintaining a healthy lifestyle. It is critical to have an awareness of the possible manifestations and indicators of kidney disease, as well as the ability to communicate any concerns with your healthcare physician. If you take care of your kidneys, you may help guarantee that you will continue to enjoy a high level of health and well-being far into the future.

CHAPTER 2

Preventing Kidney Disease

There are a number of measures that one may take to reduce their risk of developing kidney disease, some of which are as follows:

Maintaining a healthy lifestyle: Upholding a healthy lifestyle entails a number of behavioral changes, such as consuming nutritious food, engaging in regular physical activity, giving up smoking, and cutting down on alcohol intake.

Controlling blood pressure and blood sugar levels: Monitoring blood pressure and blood sugar levels and taking any necessary medication to keep them under control Both high blood pressure and high blood sugar levels can increase the risk of kidney disease, so it is essential to monitor these levels and take any medications necessary to keep them under control.

Maintaining enough hydration: Drinking a lot of water will assist the kidneys in flushing waste materials out of the body and aid to keep the kidneys in excellent condition.

Avoiding exposure to drugs and toxins that can cause kidney damage: Limiting certain medicines, such as nonsteroidal anti-inflammatory drugs (NSAIDs), as well as avoiding exposure to chemicals, such as lead and cadmium, may help reduce the risk of kidney damage that can be caused by pharmaceuticals and pollutants.

Regular check-ups: Checkups on a regular basis Having checkups on a regular basis with a healthcare practitioner may assist in the early detection of kidney disease, which in turn enables quick treatment and the prevention of major consequences.

Early treatment of urinary tract infections (UTIs): Urinary tract infections (also known as UTIs) need to be treated as soon as possible because, if left untreated for an extended period of time, they can cause permanent damage to the kidneys. For this reason, it is critical to seek medical attention as soon as possible if you experience symptoms of a UTI.

Treatment of the underlying illnesses: Treating the underlying disorders, such as diabetes and high blood pressure, may be an effective way to help avoid the development of kidney disease.

In order to keep one's kidneys in excellent condition and to forestall the onset of renal disease, one must make it a priority to take the necessary preventative measures. It is vital to share your worries about your risk for kidney disease with your healthcare professional if you are worried about your likelihood of developing the condition.

Alterations to One's Way of Life to Improve Kidney Health

Alterations to one's way of life, such as those listed below, may be helpful in preserving kidney health and warding off the onset of renal disease.

Eating a healthy diet: Consuming a diet that is rich in fruits, vegetables, and whole grains while containing a moderate amount of salt, sugar, and unsaturated fats is an example of a diet that is considered to be healthy.

Participating in regular physical activity: Participating in regular physical activity may assist in the maintenance of a healthy weight, the regulation of blood pressure and blood sugar levels, and a reduction in the risk of renal disease. Because high blood pressure, also known as hypertension, may play a role in the advancement of kidney failure, another important step for you to take is to make adjustments to your lifestyle in order to help decrease your blood pressure. If it is medically required, your doctor may suggest that you shed a few pounds in order to attain a healthy weight, which is something that may be accomplished in part via physical activity. Even if you are already at a healthy weight, you may still benefit from mild exercise in the form of lowering and keeping your blood pressure under control. Make it a goal to get at least 30 minutes of exercise every day, preferably engaging in low-impact activities such as walking, yoga, bicycling, running, or anything else that your physician has given the green light for.

Putting an end to one's smoking habit: Given that smoking is linked to an increased risk of kidney disease, as well as a plethora of other health issues, putting an end to one's smoking habit is an essential step in maintaining excellent kidney health. If you currently smoke cigarettes or use any other kind of tobacco, you should make every effort to stop as soon as you can. Even though this might be a challenging task for anybody, it is very necessary for maintaining the health of your kidneys. The blood supply to vital organs such as the kidneys is reduced when a person smokes, which may make the renal disease more severe.

Limiting alcohol consumption: Consumption of alcohol should be kept at a reasonable level since excessive alcohol consumption is associated with an increased risk of renal disease as well as many other health concerns. For this reason, it is essential to keep the consumption of alcohol at a moderate level.

Keeping your body hydrated: Consuming a large quantity of water may assist the kidneys in flushing waste items out of the body and help maintain healthy renal function.

Managing stress: Because chronic stress can increase the risk of kidney disease, in addition to the risk of many other health problems, it is important to manage stress in a healthy way, such as through exercise, relaxation techniques, or therapy. Managing stress in a healthy way can be accomplished.

Getting enough sleep: Sleep is vital for general health and well-being, and getting enough sleep may help minimize the chance of developing kidney disease. Sleeping for the recommended amount of time each night

Making these modifications to your way of life may assist in preserving kidney health and aid in warding off the development of renal disease. It is vital to share your worries about your risk for kidney disease with your healthcare professional if you are worried about your likelihood of developing the condition.

The Role of Diet and Nutrition in Maintaining Healthy Kidneys

It is essential to consume a diet that is both well-balanced and healthful in order to keep one's kidneys in excellent condition and to forestall the development of renal disease. **Limiting Salt Consumption:** Consuming an excessive amount of salt may cause blood pressure to rise, which in turn puts additional stress on the kidneys and raises the chance of developing renal disease. Keeping your salt intake to a reasonable level is one of the best things you can do for your kidneys. It is suggested that individuals limit their daily consumption of salt to no more than 2,300 milligrams.

Limiting protein intake: Consumption of protein should be restricted since eating a diet rich in protein may increase the strain on the kidneys and the likelihood of developing renal disease. Consuming a reasonable quantity of protein, such as the recommended daily requirement of 0.8 grams of protein per kilogram of body weight, is something that is strongly suggested.

Limiting Sugar Intake: Consuming a lot of sugar may lead to higher levels of blood sugar, which can in turn raise the chance of developing kidney disease. It is advisable to cut down on sugar consumption and choose natural foods that are not sweetened whenever it is feasible.

Selecting Fats That Are Good for You: The likelihood of developing kidney disease is exacerbated by the consumption of unhealthy lipids such as saturated and trans fats. It is advised that you choose healthy fats, such as the unsaturated fats that may be found in fatty fish, nuts, and seeds.

Consuming a wide range of fruits and vegetables: Fruits and vegetables include a wealth of vitamins, minerals, and antioxidants, all of which may contribute to the maintenance of healthy kidneys. If you want to acquire a broad range of different nutrients, it is advised that you consume a variety of colored fruits and vegetables.

Maintaining enough hydration: Drinking a lot of water will assist the kidneys in flushing waste materials out of the body and aid to keep the kidneys in excellent condition. It is highly advised that one consumes at least eight glasses of water on a daily basis.

Before making any substantial changes to your diet, it is crucial to talk with a healthcare professional or a trained dietitian, particularly if you have kidney disease or other medical issues. They are able to give individualized dietary suggestions that are tailored to your specific requirements and the state of your health.

Pick out meals that are good for your heart as well as the rest of your body, such as fresh fruits, fresh or frozen veggies, whole grains, and dairy products that are low in fat or fat-free. Eat a balanced diet and limit your intake of added sugars and salt to improve your health. Aim to limit your daily salt intake to fewer than 2,300 milligrams. You should strive to have added sugars account for less than 10 percent of your daily calorie intake.

Advice for deciding on nutritious options while shopping for food

- When cooking, use a combination of spices in place of salt.
- When making your pizza, choose vegetable toppings like spinach, broccoli, and peppers instead of meat.
- Instead of frying meat, poultry, or fish, you could try baking or broiling them instead.
- Do not serve items with sauce or additional fats on top.
- Make an effort to choose foods that have either very little or no added sugar.
- Start with whole milk and work your way down to milk with 2% fat until you are drinking and cooking

with fat-free (skim) or low-fat milk and milk products. This process should be done gradually.

- Eat meals that are made from whole grains on a daily basis. Some examples of whole-grain foods are whole wheat, brown rice, oats, and whole-grain maize. Brown rice should be used in place of white rice in all home-cooked meals as well as while eating out. Whole-grain bread should be used for toast and sandwiches.

- Be sure to read the labels on food. Pick meals that are low in saturated fats, trans fats, cholesterol, salt (sodium), and added sugars if you want to improve your health.

- Take it easy when it's time for a snack. It takes far more time to consume a whole bag of low-fat popcorn than it does a single piece of cake. Instead of sipping orange juice, you should peel an orange and consume it.

- Attempt to maintain a written record of everything you consume for one week.

Monitoring and Managing Chronic Health Diseases

Chronic health conditions such as diabetes and high blood pressure may raise the risk of developing kidney disease. If you have a tendency to overeat or consume meals that are heavy in fat or calories, this tool can help you detect when you are doing so. As a result, it is essential to keep a close eye on and properly treat these disorders in order to preserve healthy kidneys. If you have chronic kidney disease (CKD), you have the ability to take precautions to safeguard your kidneys from further injury. It is in your best interest to get a diagnosis of renal illness as quickly as possible. It is possible that the measures you take to protect your kidneys from injury may also assist avoid heart disease and will enhance your health in general. Making these adjustments while you are not experiencing any symptoms may be challenging for you, but it will be well worth the effort. The following is a list of some advice that may be used to monitor and manage chronic health conditions:

Regular Monitoring: It is essential to do routine monitoring of chronic health disorders, such as blood sugar levels in diabetics, in order to be certain that the illnesses are under control. Your healthcare professional will be able to provide you with advice about the frequency with which you should check your condition. Maintaining proper management of your blood pressure is the single most critical thing you can do to address renal disease. Your kidneys are susceptible to injury if you have high blood pressure. Maintaining a blood pressure that is at, or lower than, the target established by your healthcare professional is one of the best ways to preserve your kidneys. The aim for blood pressure should be less than 140/90 mm Hg for the majority of individuals. Develop a strategy for achieving your desired blood pressure levels in collaboration with your primary care physician. You may be able to lower your blood pressure by stopping smoking, engaging in physical activity, getting an adequate amount of sleep, eating meals that are heart-healthy, and reducing the amount of salt you consume, as well as taking your medications exactly as directed.

Medicine Management: If you have a health condition that is chronic, you may be required to take the medication in order to effectively manage your condition. It is essential to take your medicine exactly as directed and to keep your doctor informed of any changes in your health condition or any adverse effects the drug may cause. Some helpful hints for managing your medications are provided below.

When you pick up your next prescription or purchase an over-the-counter drug or supplement, be sure to ask the pharmacist how the product may: impact your kidneys; interact with other medications you take; or influence both of these things.

You should only have your prescriptions filled at a single drugstore or pharmacy chain. This will allow the pharmacist to: maintain track of your medications and supplements; check for any hazardous interactions.

Maintain an accurate record of the medications and supplements you use: Your wallet should always have an up-to-date list of all the medications and supplements you take. At each and every one of your doctor's appointments, you should bring either your list or all of the bottles containing your medications.

Maintaining A Healthy Lifestyle: Modifying one's lifestyle to include healthier choices, such as consuming a healthy diet, engaging in regular physical activity, giving up smoking, and finding healthy ways to deal with stress, can assist in the management of chronic health conditions and lower one's risk of developing kidney disease.

Create A Food Plan Together with The Help of a Dietician.

You may help preserve your kidneys, meet your blood pressure and blood glucose goals, and avoid or postpone health issues caused by the renal disease by paying attention to what you put in your body and what you drink.

If your kidney condition is becoming worse, you may need to make further adjustments to the foods and beverages you consume. A nutritionist who is knowledgeable about renal illness may work with you to develop a meal plan that takes into account your preferences and includes foods that are good for you while also being satisfying to eat. If you want to eat better, you should try to do as much of your food preparation and cooking from scratch as possible.

Medical nutrition therapy refers to the practice of receiving dietary advice from a qualified dietitian with the intention of achieving specific health or medical objectives (MNT).

MNT may be covered by your health insurance if you have diabetes or renal disease and a recommendation from your primary care physician to get the treatment. MNT is included in Medicare's coverage if you are eligible for the program.

Your primary care physician or another member of your healthcare team may be able to recommend a dietician to you. You may also discover a registered dietitian by going to the website of the Academy of Nutrition and Dietetics and following the link provided there. Learn how to eat properly to manage your CKD by working closely with your dietician.

Keeping An Eye on Kidney Function: If you have a disease that is chronic, it is essential to get your kidney function checked on a regular basis so that your doctor can monitor your kidney health. The frequency with which you should have these tests might be recommended to you by your healthcare professional.

Treatment At an Early Stage: In the event that kidney disease occurs, receiving therapy as soon as possible may impede the illness's course and improve results. The early detection of kidney disease by routine monitoring and treatment of chronic health issues may help save patients' lives.

It is essential to have continuous communication with your healthcare practitioner in order to monitor and manage any chronic diseases you may have. They will assess your kidney health and give individualized advice as well as assistance in order to assist you in preserving your kidney health and warding off the development of renal disease.

CHAPTER 3

Treatment Options

Options Available for the Treatment of Kidney Disease The treatment options available for kidney conditions vary depending on the kind, severity, and primary cause of the disease. The following is a list of typical treatments that may be used for kidney disease:

Medication: To treat the underlying condition that leads to kidney diseases such as high blood pressure, diabetes, or an infection, a doctor may give medication to the patient. Medication may also be administered to address symptoms and problems of kidney disease, such as anemia and fluid accumulation. Symptoms and complications of kidney disease include:

Dialysis: When the kidneys are no longer able to remove waste materials from the blood, a procedure known as dialysis may be used to accomplish this task. Dialysis may be broken down into two primary subtypes: hemodialysis and peritoneal dialysis. Peritoneal dialysis may be done at home, but hemodialysis must be done in a specialized facility called a dialysis center.

A Kidney Transplant: is a medical operation that includes the replacement of a damaged or diseased kidney with a healthy kidney donated by a donor. People who have reached the terminal stage of the renal disease often benefit most from a kidney transplant as their therapy of choice.

Lifestyle changes: Modifications to one's way of life, such as adopting a healthier diet, engaging in regular physical activity, giving up smoking, and learning to better manage stress, may assist in the management of the symptoms and consequences of kidney disease. Alterations to one's way of life may not only enhance general health but also reduce the advancement of renal disease.

Care That Is Supportive: Care that is supportive may involve steps to treat symptoms and consequences of renal disease. These may include control of fluid and electrolyte balances, as well as management of anemia. Counseling and support groups are two examples of the types of mental and emotional well-being-bolstering activities that may be included in supportive care. It is essential to have a solid working relationship with your healthcare practitioner in order to develop the most appropriate treatment plan for your specific requirements and current state of health. They are able to provide individualized guidance and assistance in order to assist you in the management of your renal illness and in the preservation of your overall health.

Medication and treatment options for kidney disease include the following

The drugs and treatments that are administered for kidney illness are different based on the kind of disease and the degree to which it has progressed. The following are examples of common drugs and treatments:

Medication For Blood Pressure: Medication for high blood pressure, such as angiotensin-converting enzyme inhibitors (ACE inhibitors) and angiotensin receptor blockers (ARBs), is often used to control high blood pressure and to decrease the course of renal disease.

Medications For Diabetes: Diabetes treatments include the following: Metformin and insulin are two examples of diabetes medications that may be provided to patients in order to control their blood sugar levels, therefore preventing or treating diabetic kidney damage.

Treatments For Anemia Include: Anemia is a frequent consequence of kidney illness, and drugs like erythropoietin (EPO), which may increase the generation of red blood cells, may be recommended to patients in order to treat the condition.

Phosphorus binders: Phosphorus binders are drugs that assist to decrease the amounts of phosphorus in the blood, which is a frequent issue in kidney disease. Phosphorus levels in the blood are a major problem in kidney illness.

Vitamin And Mineral Supplements: Vitamin and mineral supplements, such as vitamin D and calcium, may be administered to patients with renal disease in order to treat nutritional deficiencies that may develop as a result of the illness.

Antibiotics: Antibiotics In order to manage infections, which are frequent consequences that may arise from renal disease, antibiotics are sometimes recommended.

Pain Meds: A physician may recommend pain drugs in order to help patients manage the pain and suffering caused by renal disease.

Dialysis: Dialysis is a treatment that removes waste products from the blood when the kidneys are unable to do so on their own. This is done via the process of dialysis.

It is important to have a good working relationship with your healthcare practitioner in order to establish which drugs and treatments are most appropriate for your unique requirements and current state of health. They are able to provide individualized guidance and assistance in order to assist you in the management of your renal illness and in the preservation of your overall health.

The Benefits and Drawbacks of Kidney Transplantation

The surgical replacement of a diseased or damaged kidney with a healthy kidney obtained from a donor is the process that is referred to as a kidney transplant. A kidney transplant is a surgical procedure that involves implanting a healthy kidney, either from a live or dead donor, into a patient whose own kidneys are no longer able to perform their intended functions. The kidneys are a pair of bean-shaped organs that are situated on each side of the spine right below the rib cage. Each one is about the size of a closed hand. Their primary responsibility is to act as a filter, removing waste, minerals, and moisture from the blood in addition to creating urine in the process. People who have reached the end stage of renal disease may be candidates for a kidney transplant, which is a therapy option that has the potential to save their lives.

Why it is carried out

In the case of renal failure, a kidney transplant is often preferred over a lifetime of dialysis therapy as the treatment of choice. Chronic kidney disease or end-stage renal disease may be treated with a kidney transplant, which can not only make you feel better but also extend your life.

When compared with dialysis, kidney transplantation is linked with a higher quality of life, lower risk of mortality, fewer limits on nutritional intake, and lower overall cost of care.

Preemptive kidney transplantation is a technique in which a patient receives a transplanted kidney before reaching the point where they need dialysis treatment. This may be beneficial for certain patients.

A dialysis is a treatment option for persons who have renal failure; however, a kidney transplant may pose more risks for certain patients. The following are some of the medical conditions that might prohibit you from receiving a kidney transplant:

- Advanced age
- Severe heart disease
- Active or recently treated cancer
- Dementia or poorly controlled mental illness
- Abuse of alcohol or drugs
- Any other factor that could affect the ability to safely undergo the procedure and take the medications required after a transplant to prevent organ rejection.

Living-donor kidney transplantation is a possibility since the replacement of two failing kidneys only requires one kidney to be given by the patient. In the event that a suitable live donor is not available, your name may be added to a waiting list for a kidney transplant so that you might get a kidney from a donor who has passed away.

The length of time you have to wait for an organ from a dead donor depends on the degree to which you match or are compatible with the donor, the amount of time you have spent on dialysis and on the transplant waitlist, and the likelihood of your survival after the transplant. Some individuals find a suitable partner within a few months, while others may have to wait many years. When determining whether or not a kidney transplant is the best option for you, you must take into account the benefits as well as the drawbacks of this medical procedure.

Pros

Increased satisfaction with life: People who have reached the end stage of renal disease may see a significant improvement in their quality of life after undergoing a kidney transplant that is successful. In most cases, individuals who have had a kidney transplant enjoy an increase in their levels of energy, an improvement in their appetite, and a reduction in symptoms such as fluid accumulation, edema, and exhaustion.

Increased lifespan: Lifespan extension Patients who have reached the terminal stage of renal disease have a better chance of living longer if they get a kidney transplant. People who have kidney transplants often live longer and have a better outlook than those who continue to get dialysis treatment for their condition.

Freedom: A kidney transplant may boost a patient's level of independence while also reducing the frequency of dialysis treatments that are required. People who get a kidney transplant are able to resume a more regular schedule and many of the activities they loved doing before the start of renal illness. This allows them to live healthier and more fulfilling lives.

Cons

Surgery risks: Hazards associated with surgery Kidney transplantation is a significant medical treatment that entails risks associated with surgery. These risks include the possibility of bleeding, infection, and rejection of the transplanted kidney.

The lifetime of immunosuppressant drugs: Immunosuppressant medication for life Patients who have had kidney transplant surgery is required to take immunosuppressant medication for the rest of their lives in order to prevent their bodies from rejecting the donated kidney. These medications may have adverse effects, and there is a possibility that they can raise the risk of developing certain infections and malignancies.

Waiting for a donor: People who have renal illness may be placed on a transplant waiting list for a number of years before a kidney that is appropriate for transplantation becomes available. The wait for a suitable donor kidney may be a lengthy process.

Rejection of the transplanted kidney: the recipient's immune system has the potential to reject the kidney that has been transplanted. It is possible for this to happen even while immunosuppressant medicines are being used, and it may result in the need for further therapies or a return to dialysis.

Before settling on a choice, it is important to have a candid conversation with your healthcare professional about the benefits and drawbacks of kidney transplantation, as well as to thoughtfully explore all of your available alternatives. Your healthcare professional will be able to assist you in determining the treatment plan that is most appropriate for your unique requirements and current state of health.

Dialysis: An Overview of the Available Options

When the kidneys are no longer able to remove waste materials from the blood, a procedure called dialysis may be necessary. People who have a renal disease that has progressed to its last stage and need to have their blood cleansed on a regular basis to maintain their health are often candidates for dialysis. Patients whose kidneys have failed often need dialysis as a therapy option. When a person has renal failure, their kidneys are unable to filter blood as effectively as they normally would. As a direct consequence of this, waste products and poisons accumulate in your circulation. The kidneys are responsible for filtering waste materials and excess fluid from the circulation, although dialysis may perform this function instead.

Who really needs to get dialysis?

A dialysis is a treatment option that may be necessary for patients who have reached the end stage of kidney disease (ESRD). Damage to the kidneys, which may lead to renal disease, can be caused by trauma and illnesses such as high blood pressure, diabetes, and lupus.

There are certain persons who are prone to developing renal issues for no apparent cause. Kidney failure may be a chronic ailment, or it can develop quickly (acutely) after a serious illness or accident. Either way, it can have a significant impact on a person's quality of life. As you get well, this particular kind of renal failure can go away.

Kidney disease progresses via five distinct phases. When your kidney illness has progressed to stage 5, medical professionals will diagnose you as having the end-stage renal disease (ESRD), also known as kidney failure. Around 10–15 percent of the kidneys' typical function is being carried out by the time this moment arrives. To continue living, you could need kidney transplantation or dialysis treatment. While they wait for a transplant, some patients have to go through the process of dialysis. Dialysis may be broken down into two primary subtypes: hemodialysis and peritoneal dialysis.

Hemodialysis

A therapy known as hemodialysis involves passing the patient's blood through an artificial kidney machine in order to cleanse it. Hemodialysis is conducted at a hospital or a clinic that specializes in the procedure, and each session normally lasts between three and four hours. Sessions occur three times each week.

What comes first, the hemodialysis or the dialysate?

In order to make it simpler to reach the bloodstream during hemodialysis, a brief surgical procedure will be performed on you before you begin treatment. It's possible that:

A surgeon will join an artery and a vein in your arm if you have an Arteriovenous Fistula, also known as an AV fistula.

Arteriovenous graft (AV graft): Your surgeon will use a graft (a soft, hollow tube) to link the artery and vein if the artery and vein are too short to connect directly.

Because AV fistulas and grafts increase the linked artery and vein, access to dialysis is simplified as a result of their use.

They also assist in the acceleration of blood flow both inside and outside the body.

In the event that you need immediate dialysis, your healthcare professional may insert a catheter (a thin tube) into a vein in your neck, chest, or leg in order to give you temporary access.

Your healthcare professional will instruct you on how to avoid getting infections in your graft or fistula. If you like, this provider may also instruct you on how to do hemodialysis in the comfort of your own home.

What takes place throughout the process of hemodialysis?

During hemodialysis, the dialysis machine will do the following:

• It will withdraw blood from a needle that is inserted into your arm.

• Passes the blood via a filter inside the dialyzer, which transfers waste into the solution that is used for dialysis. This cleaning solution is made up of water, salt, and a few additional components as well.

• Through a separate needle inserted in your arm, the filtered blood is reintroduced to your body.

• Keeps an eye on your blood pressure in order to regulate the rate at which blood enters and leaves your body.

What comes next following hemodialysis treatment?

During their hemodialysis treatment or soon thereafter, some patients have low blood pressure. It is possible that you may feel queasy, lightheaded, or faint.

Other potential adverse effects of hemodialysis include:

- discomfort in the chest or back.
- Headaches.
- Skin that is itchy.
- Muscle cramps.
- Restless legs syndrome.

Hemodialysis can be performed at a dialysis center or hospital, which can be convenient for people who do not have access to peritoneal dialysis equipment or who prefer not to perform dialysis at home.

Pros

Flexibility: Hemodialysis can be performed at a dialysis center or hospital. This can be convenient for people who do not want to perform dialysis at home.

Individualization: Because hemodialysis may be adapted to the specific requirements of the patient, it is a treatment option that may be helpful for those who have many chronic medical issues.

Cons

Time commitment: Hemodialysis requires a major time commitment since each session normally lasts between three and four hours, and patients must undergo the procedure three times each week.

Access to equipment: People who reside in rural or distant places may have a more difficult time gaining access to necessary medical equipment since their distance from a dialysis facility or hospital may be greater than in other areas.

Cost: The cost of hemodialysis might be prohibitive for some patients since the treatment often necessitates visits to the dialysis clinic, which can be a costly endeavor in and of itself.

Peritoneal Dialysis

Peritoneal dialysis is a therapy that filters waste materials from the blood by introducing a specific solution into the belly and working its way around the abdominal cavity. Dialysis via the peritoneal cavity may be done at home, albeit the process normally takes several hours each day.

What Occurs Prior to Beginning Peritoneal Dialysis?

A simple surgical procedure will need to be performed on you around three weeks before you begin peritoneal dialysis treatment. A catheter is a flexible, thin tube that is threaded into the abdominal cavity and into the peritoneum by a surgeon. This catheter is designed to remain in its position forever. You will get instruction from a medical professional on how to administer peritoneal dialysis at home as well as how to avoid infections at the catheter site.

What Occurs During the Procedure Called Peritoneal Dialysis?

When doing peritoneal dialysis, you will need to do the following:

- Attach the catheter to one of the branches of a Y-shaped tube. This tube is connected to a bag that contains the solution used in dialysis. The peritoneal cavity is reached by the solution as it travels via the tube and the catheter.
- After about ten minutes, after the bag has been emptied, disconnect the tube and the catheter.
- Put the cap back on the catheter.
- Continue with your normal activities while the dialysis solution within the peritoneal cavity takes waste and surplus fluids from the body. This will take some time, so be patient. This procedure may take sixty to ninety minutes to complete.
- Take off the cap that's on the catheter, and then use the other arm of the Y-shaped tube to pour the fluid into a bag that's been well-cleaned and is empty.

- Perform these instructions as many times per day as you feel comfortable with. You spend the night with the solution still present in your stomach.

Nighttime peritoneal dialysis treatment is more convenient for certain patients. A device known as a cycler is used in automated peritoneal dialysis, and it is designed to pump fluid into and out of the body while the patient is asleep.

What Occurs Following a Peritoneal Dialysis Session?

It's possible that the fluid in your stomach is making you feel bloated or too full. The therapy itself is not painful, despite the fact that it may feel unpleasant. When your stomach is full of fluid, it may protrude farther than normal from your body.

Pros

Convenience: Peritoneal dialysis may be done at home, which can be advantageous for persons who do not have access to hemodialysis equipment or who want to do dialysis in the comfort of their own homes. Convenience is also a benefit for people who are unable to tolerate the side effects of hemodialysis.

Flexibility: Peritoneal dialysis is advantageous for persons who have hectic schedules since it may be carried out at any hour of the day or night, making it a flexible treatment option.

Cons

Equipment and supplies: It is necessary to have access to specialized equipment and supplies in order to perform peritoneal dialysis. These items may be rather pricey and may not be covered by insurance policies.

Time commitment: Peritoneal dialysis normally takes place over the course of several hours every day, which may be a sizable commitment of one's time.

It is crucial to have a conversation with your healthcare practitioner about the many possibilities for dialysis in order to select the optimal treatment plan for your specific requirements and current state of health. Your healthcare practitioner will be able to give you individualized advice and assistance in order to assist you in managing your kidney disease and preserving your general health.

CHAPTER 4

Coping with Kidney Disease

Living with kidney disease may be difficult, therefore it is vital to discover methods to deal with the illness's physical, emotional, and practical demands. Finding a means to live with the disease's needs might be difficult. The following is a list of suggestions for dealing with kidney disease:

Get the upper hand: You should become knowledgeable about your condition and actively participate in the management of your health care. You may find that you have a greater sense of control as well as a reduction in tension and anxiety as a result of this.

Make connections with other people: Make an effort to get emotional support and aid with practical matters from family, friends, or support groups. It may be reassuring to talk to other people who have faced similar difficulties, and doing so can bring helpful new perspectives.

Stay active: Maintaining an active lifestyle is important since getting enough regular exercise may help enhance energy levels, improve mood, and decrease stress. Pick out pursuits that are beneficial to your well-being without sacrificing your sense of fun.

Maintain a balanced diet: The advancement of renal disease may be slowed down by eating a healthy, well-balanced diet that is low in sodium, potassium, and phosphorus. Consult with a trained dietitian in order to develop a meal plan that caters to your specific dietary requirements.

Practice stress management: Long-term stress may have a detrimental effect on one's physical health. To better manage stress and enhance one's general health, it might be helpful to practice relaxation methods such as yoga, meditation, or deep breathing.

Discover your significance and your purpose: Participate in pursuits such as volunteer work, hobbies, or spiritual practices that make you happy and give you a sense of accomplishment. Pursuing experiences that are significant to oneself may help one keep a cheerful attitude while also reducing emotions of tension and worry.

It is important that you identify the methods of coping that are most successful for you and that you look for help from medical experts, family members, and friends. It is vital to keep in mind that kidney disease is a condition that lasts a lifetime, and it is crucial to discover appropriate strategies to manage it over the long term.

Managing Physical and Emotional Symptoms

Living with kidney illness may have a substantial influence on a person's physical and mental well-being, therefore it is important to learn how to effectively manage the symptoms of this condition. The discomfort and difficulty in managing the symptoms of renal disease may be emotionally demanding, and coping with the difficulties presented by the illness itself can be tough to do. It is essential to treat the physical as well as the psychological symptoms of renal disease in order to live a normal life.

Signs and Symptoms in the Body

Fatigue: Fatigue is a frequent symptom of renal illness, and it may make it difficult to carry out activities of daily living. In order to assist improve energy levels, it is important to try to have a good sleep pattern and to participate in physical exercise.

Nausea and vomiting: Nausea and vomiting are two symptoms that are often seen in patients who suffer from renal disease. Talk to your primary care physician about the possibility of taking medication to help ease these symptoms.

Pain: A common sign of kidney illness is pain, which may manifest itself in the back, sides, or belly. Have a discussion with your primary care physician about possible pain medicines and other treatment options.

Accumulation of fluid: Accumulation of fluid, also known as edema, is a typical sign of renal illness. In order to prevent further accumulation of fluid, your physician may suggest that you take diuretics.

Changes in urine output: Alterations in the amount of urine passed Changes in the amount of urine passed may be an indication of renal disease. Maintain a record of your urine output and discuss any changes with your attending physician.

Symptoms Relating to Emotions

Depression: Having a chronic ailment, such as renal disease, might make one more susceptible to developing depression. Have a conversation with your primary care physician about participating in therapy or support groups that may assist in the management of depression.

Anxiety: Living with a chronic disease often triggers feelings of anxiety in those affected by it. Make an effort to get your stress under control by practicing relaxation methods such as yoga, meditation, or deep breathing.

Difficulty with social interactions: Dealing with renal illness may make it challenging to maintain social ties, particularly if the patient is also dealing with depression or anxiety. If you need emotional support, reaching out to family, friends, or support groups may help.

It is essential to have a conversation with your healthcare practitioner about any symptoms you may be having and to get treatment for any conditions that may be present. When you are living with a chronic disease, it is vital to keep in mind that it is normal to have physical and emotional ups and downs and that it is equally necessary to take care of both your physical and mental health.

Support Systems for Patients and Caregivers

Living with kidney disease may be a stressful experience, and having support systems in place can be vital to managing both the physical and emotional symptoms of the condition. Support services are available for both patients and caregivers. Patients and caregivers alike have access to a wide variety of services that may assist in the management of the difficulties associated with renal disease.

Patients

Support groups: Patients who participate in support groups have the chance to interact with people who are coping with issues that are comparable to their own. Emotional support, knowledge, and sound counsel may all be found in plenty via participation in support groups.

Patient advocacy organizations: Groups that advocate for patients offer patients and their family's information, resources, and emotional support via the work of patient advocacy organizations. These groups also have the ability to advocate for people on crucial matters pertaining to renal illness.

Online resources: Websites, discussion boards, and groups on various social media platforms are just some of the internet tools that are readily accessible to patients and the members of their families. These sites may provide information, support, and the opportunity to connect with people who are also coping with renal illness.

Caregivers

Support groups for carers: Support groups for caregivers offer a chance for caregivers to connect with others who are going through similar struggles. Emotional support, as well as guidance and information, may all be provided via support groups.

Caregiver advocacy organizations: Groups that advocate for carers are known as caregiver advocacy organizations. These organizations provide caregivers with information, resources, and support. These organizations may also advocate for caregivers on crucial topics relating to renal illness via their various programs and services.

Respite care: Caregiver stress may be temporarily alleviated by the provision of respite care, which enables the caregiver to take a break and replenish their energy reserves. Family members, friends, or even paid carers might step in to offer temporary relief for primary caregivers.

It is crucial for patients as well as caregivers to look for assistance and services that will assist them in coping with the difficulties that come along with renal illness. Keep in mind that you are not dealing with this situation on your alone and that there are a lot of individuals and organizations who are willing to assist you.

How to Keep a Positive Attitude Despite Difficult Circumstances

The experience of living with kidney illness may be trying at times, but it is possible to have a good view despite the challenges involved. The following are some suggestions that might help you keep a happy outlook:

Focus on what you can control: Concentrate on the things that are within your power: Even though renal illness could make certain elements of your life more difficult, it is essential to put your attention on the things you are able to manage, such as your food, your exercise routine, and your prescription schedule.

Get in touch with other people: Making connections with other people who are experiencing similar difficulties may give a source of support, encouragement, and inspiration. Think about becoming a member of a support group or establishing connections with people via the use of internet tools.

Keep yourself active: Maintaining an active lifestyle and doing regular exercise may help improve both your mood and your general health and well-being. Talk to your primary care provider about the kinds of physical activities that are most appropriate for your condition.

Practice gratitude: Maintaining a good attitude may be assisted by developing an attitude of thankfulness and concentrating on the favorable parts of one's life. Keep a notebook in which you list the things for which you are grateful, or make it a point to concentrate on the positive aspects of your life on a daily basis.

Seek the assistance of a professional: If you are having trouble dealing with emotions of sadness or anxiety, you might think about seeking the assistance of a professional. Support, skills for coping, and techniques for managing stress and emotions may be provided by a therapist or counselor, among other things.

It is essential to have in mind that people from all walks of life face difficulties and failures, but that it is also within one's power to keep a positive view in spite of such problems. It is possible to live a life that is meaningful and rewarding even while dealing with renal illness provided one has access to the appropriate support and resources.

CHAPTER 5

Managing the Financial Impact of Kidney Disease

Kidney illness may have a substantial effect on a person's finances since it often necessitates the use of pricey treatments and drugs. In addition, people who have renal illness may be required to miss work, which may result in a loss of revenue for the patient. The financial burden of the renal disease will be discussed in this chapter, along with advice on how to manage it.

Gaining an understanding of the expenses associated with renal disease: It is essential to have a thorough understanding of the costs involved with renal illness, which may include the expenses incurred due to treatments, drugs, and income loss.

Coverage Under Insurance: The financial effect of renal illness may be managed in part by taking steps such as being knowledgeable about your insurance coverage and the services it provides. Patients could be qualified for several kinds of insurance, such as private insurance, Medicare, or Medicaid, depending on their circumstances.

Financial Assistance Programs: There are a variety of financial support programs that are available to patients and their families in order to assist them in managing the expenditures that are associated with renal disease. Patients can be eligible for financial support via government programs, patient advocacy groups, or medication corporations.

Managing Expenses and Creating a Budget: Creating a budget and keeping expenditures under control are two essential steps in the process of mitigating the monetary effects of renal disease. Taking care of the costs associated with therapy, drugs, and transportation is an example of what this entails.

Work And Financial Gain: Patients suffering from renal illness could be required to take time out of work, which would result in a decrease in income. It is essential that you be aware of all of your legal entitlements and available choices, such as flexible working arrangements and benefits for those with disabilities.

Patients and their families may help lessen the financial effect of kidney disease by being educated on the expenses associated with the condition and investigating the many alternatives available for financial aid. Keep in mind that it is important to look for assistance and services that might assist in managing the monetary effect of renal illness.

Fundraising And Community Support: Fundraising and obtaining support from the community are two ways to assist offset the financial cost of renal illness. In addition, gaining support from the community may help. Patients and their families are encouraged to investigate all of the possible avenues for fundraising, including benefit concerts, internet fundraising platforms, and community activities.

Having A Conversation with A Financial Adviser: A financial advisor may give very helpful advice and direction on the management of the monetary effects of renal illness. They are able to aid in the creation of a budget, the planning of future spending, and the investigation of potential sources of financial support.

Tax Benefits: Tax advantages Patients who suffer from renal illness are eligible for a number of tax advantages, including the opportunity to deduct medical expenses from their taxes and the credit for disabled taxpayers. Patients looking for information on the tax advantages that are available to them should seek the advice of a qualified tax expert.

Getting Your Medical Records and Bills in Order: Patients who are coping with the financial burden of renal illness may find that keeping detailed records of their medical bills and other costs is helpful. Patients should not throw away any receipts or invoices that are relevant to their medical bills, and they should also consider utilizing an application or program to keep track of their expenditures.

Seeking Support and Resources: Patients and their families should not be afraid to seek assistance and services in order to better manage the financial burden that renal disease has on their lives. Reaching out to support groups, financial experts, and organizations that advocate for patients are all examples of this strategy.

Putting Money into Activities That Are Good for Your Health: Even while the expenses of therapy and drugs might mount up quickly, it is essential to avoid cutting down on activities and investments that are beneficial to one's general health and well-being. This might involve practicing good eating habits, getting regular exercise, learning strategies to handle stress, and reaching out to friends and family for support.

Planning For the Future: Making preparations for the future It is essential to make preparations for the future, particularly when one is coping with a persistent condition such as renal disease. This might involve establishing financial objectives, writing a will, and having conversations with loved ones about end-of-life plans and preparations.

Maximizing Resources: The financial burden of renal illness may be tough for patients to handle, but there are numerous services available to assist them in doing so. However, it can be challenging to know where to begin. Patients and their families may seek out groups that advocate for patients to get advice on how to make the most of available resources, or they might consider working with a financial adviser who specializes in the management of costs associated with medical care.

Filing For Disability Benefits: Filing for disability benefits may be required for patients who are unable to work as a result of their renal illness. Filing for disability benefits is one option available to these patients. Patients should get acquainted with the qualifying conditions for disability benefits and understand the application procedure before submitting an application for these benefits.

Managing Stress: Dealing with the financial effect of renal illness may be stressful, but it is crucial to make stress-management skills a priority in order to have a healthy mental and physical balance. Exercising, practicing mindfulness, and reaching out to loved ones and friends for support are all potential components of this strategy.

Managing the financial effect that renal illness may have on a person's life can be difficult, but there are a variety of services and solutions available to assist with the problem. Patients and their families need to concentrate on making the most of the resources available to them, making preparations for the future, and preserving their general health and well-being.

The financial effect of kidney illness may be daunting; however, patients and their families can help lessen this impact by being knowledgeable about the expenses of treatment and researching the many alternatives available for financial aid. It is crucial to seek assistance and tools to assist in managing the financial effect of renal disease. At the same time, it is important to remember to maintain optimum health and well-being.

Understanding How Insurance Works: Patients who are dealing with the renal illness have a tremendous uphill battle when it comes to figuring out their insurance alternatives and navigating the insurance process. Patients should get informed about their available insurance coverage alternatives and consider collaborating with a healthcare advocate or insurance professional to assist with cost management for their treatment. Patients should do this since it is in their own best interest.

Exploring Alternative Funding Options: Investigating the availability of other sources of funding: Patients who lack health insurance or have inadequate coverage may benefit from investigating other financing sources, which may help reduce the overall cost of their care. This may include programs run by the government, resources run by communities themselves, or activities to raise money.

Establishing A Reliable Network of Support: Developing a solid support system might be of utmost importance when it comes to mitigating the monetary effects of renal illness. Patients and their families should strongly consider reaching out to support groups, patient advocacy organizations, and local communities for assistance and direction in order to maximize their chances of a positive outcome.

Maximizing Earning Potential: Managing the monetary burden of renal illness may be made easier for patients who are able to continue working by increasing their earning potential. Maximizing earning potential is an important step in this process. Patients who want to expand their earning potential should investigate the possibility of more flexible employment arrangements, possibilities to work from home, and educational alternatives that allow them to continue their education.

Seeking Legal Counsel: Seeking the advice of a lawyer might be advantageous for people who are having difficulty dealing with the financial burden of renal illness. The advice of an attorney may be invaluable when dealing with financial matters such as insurance claims, disability compensation, and other concerns.

In order to effectively manage the financial repercussions of renal illness, a comprehensive strategy that makes use of a broad variety of different tactics and resources is required. To better control the expenditures of therapy and to preserve their general health and well-being, patients and their families have to be proactive in examining all available choices and constructing robust support networks for themselves.

Developing an individualized treatment strategy

Understanding The Stages of Kidney Disease: An understanding of the phases of kidney illness the course of kidney disease may be broken down into five stages, each of which is characterized by its own unique collection of symptoms and treatment choices. Patients who have a better understanding of the phases of renal disease are in a better position to make educated choices about their treatment.

Locating Potential Providers of Care: In order to effectively manage renal illness, it is essential to find the appropriate care providers. Patients should discuss the possibility of developing a tailored treatment strategy in collaboration with a group of healthcare professionals, which may include nephrologists, primary care doctors, and specialists.

Maintaining Current Knowledge of Available Therapy Options: Patients who are able to keep up with the most recent developments in treatment alternatives may better participate in the decision-making process for their own medical care. Patients might think about participating in educational programs, keeping up with pertinent literature, and involving themselves in patient advocacy groups.

Collaborating With Care Providers: Working together with those who give care to patients suffering from renal disease may improve the quality of treatment they get for their condition by working in conjunction with other medical professionals. Patients and their care providers should engage in honest communication and the patient should take an active role in decision-making.

Keeping one's connections in a healthy state

Developing a robust support network: Developing a robust support network might be of utmost importance in order to effectively manage the psychological and financial effects of renal disease. Patients looking for assistance and direction should strongly consider getting in touch with patient advocacy organizations, support groups, and their local communities.

Keeping an open line of communication with loved ones: Keeping an open line of communication with loved ones is essential for effectively managing the effects that renal illness has on interpersonal connections. Patients need to give thought to the possibility of having forthright and open conversations about their requirements and constraints.

Seeking couples' therapy: Seeking out the services of a therapist who specializes in treating couples Patients who are already in a romantic relationship may find that seeking out the services of a therapist who specializes in treating couples can help them strengthen their relationship and support one another through the challenges of kidney disease.

Building a healthy self-image: Creating a positive image of oneself can be difficult for patients who suffer from kidney disease; however, it is essential for patients who wish to maintain healthy relationships. Patients should think about participating in self-care activities and reaching out to loved ones for help when they need it.

Taking care of the financial repercussions of kidney disease can be an overwhelming task, but it is essential to seize control of the situation and devise a strategy. Patients and their families can find peace of mind and stability despite the presence of this disease if they educate themselves regarding the costs of treatment, investigate the availability of financial assistance options, take steps to reduce expenses, and plan for the future.

CONCLUSION

Kidney illness is a complicated disorder that may have a significant effect on a person's physical health as well as their mental state and their ability to maintain their financial stability. It is very necessary to have a complete awareness of the condition, as well as its origins, risk factors, and potential treatments.

In this book, we have discussed the structure of the kidneys as well as their functions, as well as the significance of protecting renal health, and the numerous conditions that may affect kidney function. We have also discussed how to diagnose the ailment, in addition to its causes and the variables that put patients at risk for developing it.

In addition, we have explored methods for avoiding kidney disease, such as making adjustments to one's lifestyle, adhering to a balanced food and nutrition plan, and keeping an eye on and effectively managing chronic health issues. We have also discussed the many different treatment choices that are accessible to people who are afflicted with kidney disease. These alternatives include medication, therapy, dialysis, and transplantation. It is critical for patients who are dealing with kidney illness to have support networks in place since this is essential for their overall physical and mental wellness. Managing the symptoms of the condition may be difficult; however, keeping an optimistic perspective and cultivating relationships with those who have been through something similar can bring both solace and hope.

Managing renal illness, on the other hand, calls for taking a holistic approach, which involves putting equal emphasis on one's physical health, mental well-being, and financial security. Patients and their families are able to traverse this road with better confidence and hope for maximum health if they have a thorough grasp of the condition, its effects, and the many treatment and support choices available.

The Prospects for Kidney Health and Research in the Future

Those who are now coping with renal illness may continue to take heart in the progress that has been made in medical technology and research. There have been tremendous breakthroughs in the treatment and management of renal illness in recent years, and it is anticipated that this trend will continue in the foreseeable future.

The field of regenerative medicine, which aims to repair or replace damaged organs and tissues, is one of the study areas that shows a lot of promise in the future. Researchers are investigating novel methods for the regeneration of injured kidney tissue and the development of functioning replacement organs. If successful, these endeavors might completely transform the management of kidney illness.

Personalized medicine is another area of concentration, and this branch of medicine develops treatment strategies by taking an individual's unique genetic profile, lifestyle, and medical history into consideration. This strategy may result in more successful therapies that are adapted to the individual requirements of a patient, hence improving the patient's overall quality of life.

The use of artificial intelligence (AI) in the diagnosis and treatment of renal disease is yet another interesting and promising new discovery. In order to deliver more accurate diagnoses and treatment regimens, AI algorithms are able to assess enormous volumes of patient data, such as imaging, test findings, and medical history.

Taking Charge of Your Kidney Health Right This Very Minute

Although there is the reason for optimism about kidney health and research in the years to come, it is critical that you take charge of your kidney health right now. If you've already been diagnosed with kidney disease, there are a number of straightforward actions you can take to improve your quality of life and lower your chance of having the illness in the future.

Keeping up a healthy lifestyle is one of the most crucial actions that you can do. This involves maintaining a healthy lifestyle by eating a balanced diet, being active, giving up smoking, and reducing the amount of alcohol you consume. You may help lower your chance of getting kidney disease by keeping your weight at a reasonable level, managing your blood pressure and cholesterol levels, and maintaining overall good health.

The monitoring and management of any chronic health diseases that you may have, such as diabetes or high blood pressure, is another essential step that you must do. Keeping these diseases under control and minimizing the effect they have on your kidney health may be accomplished with the aid of regular checkups with your healthcare provider and by adhering to the treatment plan that they propose.

If you have been told that you have kidney disease, taking charge of your treatment and care is an additional step that should not be overlooked. Collaborate with your source of healthcare to establish a specific treatment plan, and make it a point to remain current on the most recent developments in treatments and therapies. You may also want to think about becoming a member of a support group or making connections with other patients who are going through something like this.

In conclusion, taking charge of your kidney health now may help you lower your chance of getting kidney disease and enhance the quality of your life if you have already been diagnosed with the condition. You may help assure a bright future for your kidney health by choosing to live a healthy lifestyle, monitoring and managing your health issues, and taking an active part in your treatment and care.